C000228815

My Favo

Ketogenic Air Fryer

Meals

Tasty and Affordable Ketogenic Air Fryer Recipes to Start Your Day with the Right Foot

Morgan Parry

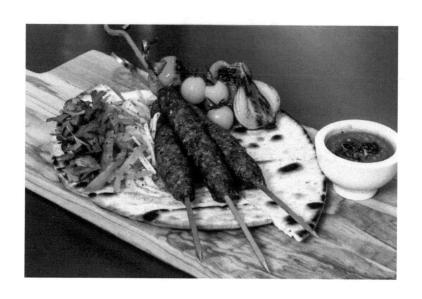

© **Copyright 2021 - All rights reserved.**

The content contained within this book may not be reproduced, duplicated or transmitted without direct written permission from the author or the publisher.

Under no circumstances will any blame or legal responsibility be held against the publisher, or author, for any damages, reparation, or monetary loss due to the information contained within this book. Either directly or indirectly.

Legal Notice:

This book is copyright protected. This book is only for personal use. You cannot amend, distribute, sell, use, quote or paraphrase any part, or the content within this book, without the consent of the author or publisher.

Disclaimer Notice:

Please note the information contained within this document is for educational and entertainment purposes only. All effort has been executed to present accurate, up to date, and reliable, complete information. No warranties of any kind are declared or implied. Readers acknowledge that the author is not engaging in the rendering of legal, financial, medical or professional advice. The content within this book has been derived from various sources. Please consult a licensed professional before attempting any techniques outlined in this book.

By reading this document, the reader agrees that under no circumstances is the author responsible for any losses, direct or indirect, which are incurred as a result of the use of information contained within this document, including, but not limited to, — errors, omissions, or inaccuracies.

Table of Contents

Chia Bites

Prep time: 15 minutes

Cooking time: 8 minutes

Servings: 2

Ingredients:

- ½ scoop of protein powder

- 1 egg, beaten

- 3 tablespoons almond flour

- 1 oz hazelnuts, grinded

- 1 tablespoon flax meal

- 1 teaspoon Splenda

- 1 teaspoon butter, softened

- 1 teaspoon chia seeds, dried

- ¼ teaspoon ground clove

Directions:

1.   In the mixing bowl mix up protein powder, almond flour, grinded hazelnuts, flax meal, chia seeds, ground clove, and Splenda. Then add egg and butter and stir it

with the help of the spoon until you get a homogenous mixture. Cut the mixture into pieces and make 2 bites of any shape with the help of the fingertips. Preheat the air fryer to 365F. Line the air fryer basket with baking paper and put the protein bites inside.

2.   Cook them for 8 minutes.

Nutrition: calories 433, fat 35.5, fiber 7, carbs 15.6, protein 20.2

Espresso Cinnamon Cookies

Preparation time: 5 minutes

Cooking time: 15 minutes

Servings: 12

Ingredients:

- 8 tablespoons ghee, melted 1 cup almond flour

- ¼ cup brewed espresso

- ¼ cup swerve

- ½ tablespoon cinnamon powder 2 teaspoons baking powder

- 2 eggs, whisked

Directions:

1. In a bowl, mix all the ingredients and whisk well. Spread medium balls on a cookie sheet lined parchment paper, flatten them, put the cookie sheet in your air fryer and cook at 350 degrees F for 15 minutes. Serve the cookies cold.

Nutrition: calories 134, fat 12, fiber 2, carbs 4, protein 2

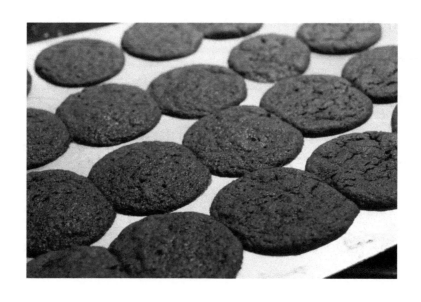

Turmeric Almond Pie

Prep time: 20 minutes

Cooking time: 35 minutes

Servings: 4

Ingredients:

- 4 eggs, beaten
- 1 tablespoon poppy seeds
- 1 teaspoon ground turmeric
- 1 teaspoon vanilla extract
- 1 teaspoon baking powder
- 1 teaspoon lemon juice
- 1 cup almond flour
- 2 tablespoons heavy cream
- ¼ cup Erythritol
- 1 teaspoon avocado oil

Directions:

1.   Put the eggs in the bowl. Add vanilla extract, baking powder, lemon juice, almond flour, heavy cream, and Erythritol. Then add avocado oil and poppy seeds. Add turmeric. With the help of the immersion blender, blend the pie batter until it is smooth. Line the air fryer cake mold with baking paper. Pour the pie batter in the cake mold. Flatten the pie surface with the help of the spatula if needed. Then preheat the air fryer to 365F. Put the cake mold in the air fryer and cook the pie for 35 minutes. When the pie is cooked, cool it completely and remove it from the cake mold. Cut the cooked pie into the servings.

Nutrition: calories 149, fat 11.9, fiber 1.2, carbs 3.8, protein 7.7

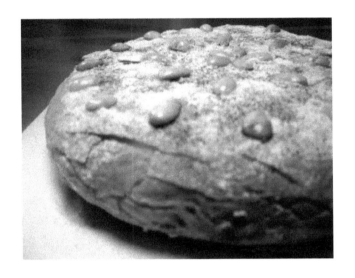

Sponge Cake

Preparation time: 5 minutes

Cooking time: 30 minutes

Servings: 8

Ingredients:

*   1 cup ricotta, soft 1/3 swerve

*   3 eggs, whisked

*   1 cup almond flour

*   7 tablespoons ghee, melted 1 teaspoon baking powder Cooking spray

Directions:

1. In a bowl, combine all the ingredients except the cooking spray and stir them very well. Grease a cake pan that fits the air fryer with the cooking spray and pour the cake mix inside. Put the pan in the fryer and cook at 350 degrees F for 30 minutes. Cool the cake down, slice and serve.

Nutrition: calories 210, fat 12, fiber 3, carbs 6, protein 9

Beef Burger

Prep time: 10 minutes

Prep time: 15 minutes

Servings: 3

Ingredients:

- ½ teaspoon salt

- 1 teaspoon cayenne pepper

- 1 teaspoon minced ginger

- 1 teaspoon minced garlic

- 2 tablespoons chives, chopped

- 6 lettuce leaves

- 10 oz ground beef

- 1 tablespoon avocado oil

- 1 teaspoon gochujang

Directions:

1.   In the shallow bowl mix up gochujang, minced ginger, minced garlic, cayenne pepper, and salt. Then mix up ground beef and churned spices mixture. Add chives and stir the ground beef mass with the help of the fork until homogenous. Preheat the air fryer to 365F. Then make 3 burgers from the ground beef mixture and put them in the air fryer. Sprinkle the burgers with avocado oil and cook for 10 minutes at 365F. Then flip the burgers on another side and cook for 5 minutes more.

Nutrition: calories195, fat 11.7, fiber 1.1, carbs 3.4, protein 18.1

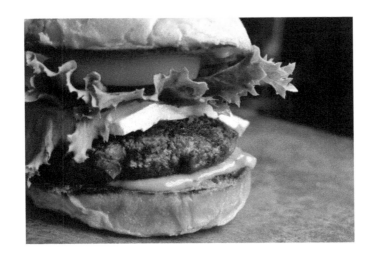

Parmesan Beef Mix

Preparation time: 5 minutes

Prep time: 20 minutes

Servings: 4

Ingredients:

- 14 ounces beef, cubed

- 7 ounces keto tomato sauce

- tablespoon chives, chopped

- tablespoons parmesan cheese, grated 1 tablespoon oregano, chopped

- 1 tablespoon olive oil

- Salt and black pepper to the taste

Directions:

1.	Grease a pan that fits the air fryer with the oil and mix all the ingredients except the parmesan. Sprinkle the parmesan on top, put the pan in the machine and cook at 380 degrees F for 20 minutes. Divide between plates and serve for lunch.

Nutrition: calories 280, fat 14, fiber 4, carbs 6, protein 15

Garlic Bread

Prep time: 10 minutes

Cooking time: 8 minutes

Servings: 4

Ingredients:

- 1 oz Mozzarella, shredded
- 2 tablespoons almond flour
- 1 teaspoon cream cheese
- ¼ teaspoon garlic powder
- ¼ teaspoon baking powder
- 1 egg, beaten
- 1 teaspoon coconut oil, melted
- ¼ teaspoon minced garlic
- 1 teaspoon dried dill
- 1 oz Provolone cheese, grated

Directions:

1.   In the mixing bowl mix up Mozzarella, almond flour, cream cheese, garlic powder, baking powder, egg, minced garlic, dried dill, and Provolone cheese. When the mixture is homogenous, transfer it on the baking paper and spread it in the shape of the bread. Sprinkle the garlic bread with coconut oil. Preheat the air fryer to 400F. Transfer the baking paper with garlic bread in the air fryer and cook for 8 minutes or until it is light brown. When the garlic bread is cooked, cut it on 4 servings and place it in the serving plates.

Nutrition: calories 155, fat 12.7, fiber 1.6, carbs 4, protein 8.3

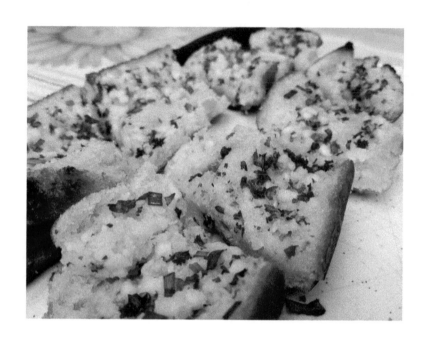

Italian Eggplant Bites

Prep time: 10 minutes

Cooking time: 10 minutes

Servings: 5

Ingredients:

- 2 medium eggplants, trimmed

- 1 tomato

- 1 teaspoon Italian seasonings

- 1 teaspoon avocado oil

- 3 oz Parmesan, sliced

Directions:

1.   Slice the eggplants on 5 slices. Then thinly slice the tomato on 5 slices. Place the eggplants in the air fryer in one layer and cook for 3 minutes from every side at 400F. After this, top the sliced eggplants with tomato, sprinkle with avocado oil and Italian seasonings. Then top the eggplants with Parmesan. Cook the meal for 4 minutes at 400F.

Nutrition: calories 116, fat 4.5, fiber 7.9, carbs 14.1, protein 7.7

Cauliflower Mash

Preparation time: 5 minutes

Cooking time: 20 minutes

Servings: 4

Ingredients:

- pounds cauliflower florets 1 teaspoon olive oil
- ounces parmesan, grated 4 ounces butter, soft
- Juice of ½ lemon
- Zest of ½ lemon, grated
- Salt and black pepper to the taste

Directions:

1. Preheated you air fryer at 380 degrees F, add the basket inside, add the cauliflower, also add the oil, rub well and cook for 20 minutes. Transfer the cauliflower to a bowl, mash well, add the rest of the ingredients, stir really well, divide between plates and serve as a side dish.

Nutrition: calories 174, fat 5, fiber 2, carbs 5, protein 8

Shrimp and Celery Salad

Prep time: 10 minutes

Cooking time: 5 minutes

Servings: 4

Ingredients:

- 3 oz chevre

- 1 teaspoon avocado oil

- ½ teaspoon dried oregano

- 8 oz shrimps, peeled

- 1 teaspoon butter, melted

- ½ teaspoon salt

- ½ teaspoon chili flakes

- 4 oz celery stalk, chopped

Directions:

1.   Sprinkle the shrimps with dried oregano and melted butter and put in the air fryer. Cook the seafood at 400F for 5 minutes. Meanwhile, crumble the chevre. Put the chopped celery stalk in the salad bowl. Add

crumbled chevre, chili flakes, salt, and avocado oil. Mix up the salad well and top it with cooked shrimps.

Nutrition: calories 158, fat 7.5, fiber 0.6, carbs 4.2, protein 17.7

Basil and Paprika Cod

Preparation time: 5 minutes

Cooking time: 15 minutes

Servings: 4

Ingredients:

- 4 cod fillets, boneless

- 1 teaspoon red pepper flakes

- ½ teaspoon hot paprika 2 tablespoon olive oil 1 teaspoon basil, dried

- Salt and black pepper to the taste

Directions:

1. In a bowl, mix the cod with all the other ingredients and toss. Put the fish in your air fryer's basket and cook at 380 degrees F for 15 minutes.

2. Divide the cod between plates and serve.

Nutrition: calories 194, fat 7, fiber 2, carbs 4, protein 12

Cajun Shrimps

Prep time: 10 minutes

Cooking time: 6 minutes

Servings: 4

Ingredients:

- 8 oz shrimps, peeled
- 1 teaspoon Cajun spices
- 1 teaspoon cream cheese
- 1 egg, beaten
- ½ teaspoon salt
- 1 teaspoon avocado oil

Directions:

1.   Sprinkle the shrimps with Cajun spices and salt. In the mixing bowl mix up cream cheese and egg, Dip every shrimp in the egg mixture. Preheat the air fryer to 400F. Place the shrimps in the air fryer and sprinkle with avocado oil. Cook the popcorn shrimps for 6 minutes. Shake them well after 3 minutes of cooking.

Nutrition: calories 88, fat 2.5, fiber 0.1, carbs 1, protein 14.4

Balsamic Cod

Preparation time: 5 minutes

Cooking time: 15 minutes

Servings: 4

Ingredients:

- 4 cod fillets, boneless
- Salt and black pepper to the taste 1 cup parmesan
- 4 tablespoons balsamic vinegar A drizzle of olive oil
- 3 spring onions, chopped

Directions:

1. Season fish with salt, pepper, grease with the oil, and coat it in parmesan. Put the fillets in your air fryer's basket and cook at 370 degrees F for 14 minutes. Meanwhile, in a bowl, mix the spring onions with salt, pepper and the vinegar and whisk. Divide the cod between plates, drizzle the spring onions mix all over and serve with a side salad.

Nutrition: calories 220, fat 12, fiber 2, carbs 5, protein 13

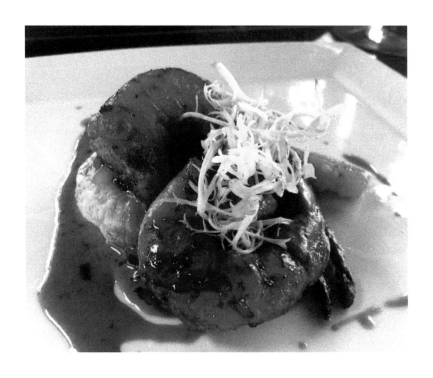

Wrapped Scallops

Prep time: 15 minutes

Cooking time: 7 minutes

Servings: 4

Ingredients:

- 1 teaspoon ground coriander
- ½ teaspoon ground paprika
- ¼ teaspoon salt
- 16 oz scallops
- 4 oz bacon, sliced
- 1 teaspoon sesame oil

Directions:

1. Sprinkle the scallops with ground coriander, ground paprika, and salt. Then wrap the scallops in the bacon slices and secure with toothpicks. Sprinkle the scallops with sesame oil. Preheat the air fryer to 400F. Put the scallops in the air fryer basket and cook them for 7 minutes.

Nutrition: calories 264, fat 13.9, fiber 0.1, carbs 3.2, protein 29.6

Cod and Sauce

Preparation time: 5 minutes

Cooking time: 15 minutes

Servings: 2

Ingredients:

- 2 cod fillets, boneless

- Salt and black pepper to the taste 1 bunch spring onions, chopped 3 tablespoons ghee, melted

Directions:

1. In a pan that fits the air fryer, combine all the ingredients, toss gently, introduce in the air fryer and cook at 360 degrees F for 15 minutes. Divide the fish and sauce between plates and serve.

Nutrition: calories 240, fat 12, fiber 2, carbs 5, protein 11

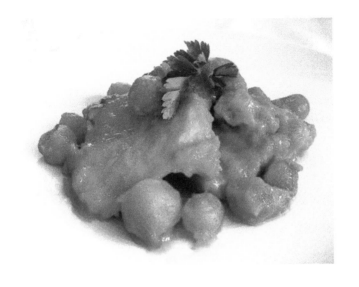

Thyme Catfish

Prep time: 10 minutes

Cooking time: 12 minutes

Servings: 4

Ingredients:

- 20 oz catfish fillet (4 oz each fillet)

- 2 eggs, beaten

- 1 teaspoon dried thyme

- ½ teaspoon salt

- 1 teaspoon apple cider vinegar

- 1 teaspoon avocado oil

- ¼ teaspoon cayenne pepper

- 1/3 cup coconut flour

Directions:

1. Sprinkle the catfish fillets with dried thyme, salt, apple cider vinegar, cayenne pepper, and coconut flour. Then sprinkle the fish fillets with avocado oil. Preheat the air fryer to 385F. Put the catfish fillets in the air fryer

basket and cook them for 8 minutes. Then flip the fish on another side and cook for 4 minutes more.

Nutrition: calories 198, fat 10.7, fiber 4.2, carbs 6.5, protein 18.3

Salmon and Creamy Chives Sauce

Preparation time: 5 minutes

Cooking time: 20 minutes

Servings: 4

Ingredients:

- 4 salmon fillets, boneless

- A pinch of salt and black pepper

- ½ cup heavy cream

- 1 tablespoon chives, chopped 1 teaspoon lemon juice

- 1 teaspoon dill, chopped 2 garlic cloves, minced

- ¼ cup ghee, melted

Directions:

1. In a bowl, mix all the ingredients except the salmon and whisk well. Arrange the salmon in a pan that fits the air fryer, drizzle the sauce all over, introduce the pan in the machine and cook at 360 degrees F for 20 minutes. Divide everything between plates and serve.

Nutrition: calories 220, fat 14, fiber 2, carbs 5, protein 12

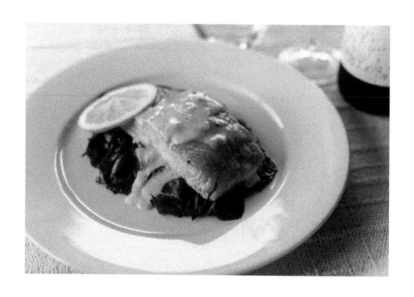

Garlic Shrimp Mix

Prep time: 10 minutes

Cooking time: 5 minutes

Servings: 3

Ingredients:

- 1-pound shrimps, peeled
- ½ teaspoon garlic powder
- ¼ teaspoon minced garlic
- 1 teaspoon ground cumin
- ¼ teaspoon lemon zest, grated
- ½ tablespoon avocado oil
- ½ teaspoon dried parsley

Directions:

1.   In the mixing bowl mix up shrimps, garlic powder, minced garlic, ground cumin, lemon zest, and dried parsley. Then add avocado oil and mix up the shrimps well. Preheat the air fryer to 400F. Put the shrimps in the preheated air fryer basket and cook for 5 minutes.

Nutrition: calories 187, fat 3, fiber 0.2, carbs 3.2, protein 34.7

Tilapia and Tomato Salsa

Preparation time: 5 minutes

Cooking time: 15 minutes

Servings: 4

Ingredients:

- 4 tilapia fillets, boneless 1 tablespoon olive oil

- A pinch of salt and black pepper 12 ounces tomatoes, chopped

- 2 tablespoons green onions, chopped

- 2 tablespoons sweet red pepper, chopped 1 tablespoon balsamic vinegar

Directions:

1. Arrange the tilapia in a baking sheet that fits the air fryer and season with salt and pepper. In a bowl, combine all the other ingredients, toss and spread over the fish. Introduce the pan in the fryer and cook at 350 degrees F for 15 minutes. Divide the mix between plates and serve.

Nutrition: calories 221, fat 12, fiber 2, carbs 5, protein 14

Lamb and Salsa

Preparation time: 5 minutes

Cooking time: 35 minutes

Servings: 4

Ingredients:

- 1 tablespoon chipotle powder

- A pinch of salt and black pepper 1 and ½ pounds lamb loin, cubed 2 tablespoons red vinegar

- 4 tablespoons olive oil 2 tomatoes, cubed

- 2 cucumbers, sliced

- 2 spring onions, chopped Juice of ½ lemon

- ¼ cup mint, chopped

Directions:

1.   Heat up a pan that fits your air fryer with half of the oil over medium-high heat, add the lamb, stir and brown for 5 minutes. Add the chipotle powder, salt pepper and the vinegar, toss, put the pan in the air fryer and cook at 380 degrees F for 30 minutes. In a bowl, mix tomatoes with cucumbers, onions, lemon juice, mint and

the rest of the oil and toss. Divide the lamb between plates, top each serving with the cucumber salsa and serve.

Nutrition: calories 284, fat 13, fiber 3, carbs 6, protein 14

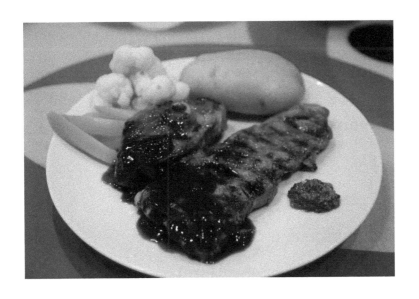

Lamb Burgers

Prep time: 15 minutes

Cooking time: 16 minutes

Servings: 2

Ingredients:

- 8 oz lamb, minced

- ½ teaspoon salt

- ½ teaspoon ground black pepper

- ½ teaspoon dried cilantro

- 1 tablespoon water

- Cooking spray

Directions:

1.   In the mixing bowl mix up minced lamb, salt, ground black pepper, dried cilantro, and water.

2.   Stir the meat mixture carefully with the help of the spoon and make 2 burgers.

3.   Preheat the air fryer to 375F.

4.   Spray the air fryer basket with cooking spray and put the burgers inside. Cook them for 8 minutes from each side.

Nutrition: calories 219, fat 8.3, fiber 0.5, carbs 1.8, protein 32

Lime Lamb Curry

Preparation time: 5 minutes

Cooking time: 35 minutes

Servings: 4

Ingredients:

- 2 tablespoons olive oil

- 1 and ½ pounds lamb meat, cubed A pinch of salt and black pepper 15 ounces tomatoes, chopped Juice of 2 limes

- teaspoon sweet paprika 1 cup beef stock

- 1-inch ginger, grated 2 hot chilies, chopped

- red bell peppers, chopped 4 garlic cloves, minced

- 2 teaspoons turmeric powder 1 tablespoon green curry paste

Directions:

1. Heat up a pan that fits your air fryer with the oil over medium heat, add the meat and brown for 5 minutes. Add the rest of the ingredients, toss, put the

pan in the fryer and cook at 380 degrees F for 30 minutes. Divide everything into bowls and serve.

Nutrition: calories 284, fat 12, fiber 3, carbs 5, protein 16

Lamb Sausages

Prep time: 25 minutes

Cooking time: 10 minutes

Servings: 4

Ingredients:

- 4 sausage links

- 12 oz ground lamb

- 1 teaspoon minced garlic

- ½ teaspoon onion powder

- 1 teaspoon dried parsley

- ½ teaspoon salt

- 1 teaspoon ghee

- ½ teaspoon ground ginger

- 1 tablespoon sesame oil

Directions:

1.   In the mixing bowl mix up ground lamb, minced garlic, onion powder, dried parsley, salt, and ground ginger. Then fill the sausage links with the ground lamb

mixture. Secure the ends of the sausages. Brush the air fryer basket with sesame oil from inside and put the sausages. Then sprinkle the sausages with ghee. Cook the lamb sausages for 10 minutes at 400F. Flip them on another side after 5 minutes of cooking.

Nutrition: calories 201, fat 10.7, fiber 0.1, carbs 0.7, protein 24

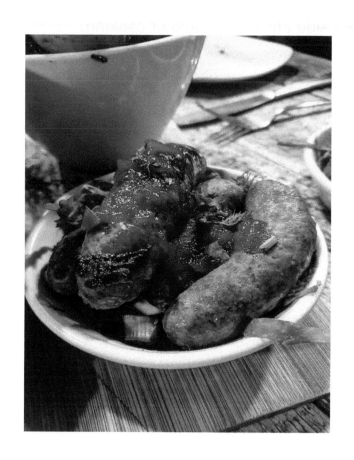

Lamb and Vinaigrette

Preparation time: 10 minutes

Cooking time: 30 minutes

Servings: 4

Ingredients:

- 4 lamb loin slices
- A pinch of salt and black pepper 3 garlic cloves, minced
- 2 teaspoons thyme, chopped 2 tablespoons olive oil
- 1/3 cup parsley, chopped
- 1/3 cup sun-dried tomatoes, chopped 2 tablespoons balsamic vinegar
- 2 tablespoons water

Directions:

1. In a blender, combine all the ingredients except the lamb slices and pulse well. In a bowl, mix the lamb with the tomato vinaigrette and toss well.

2.   Put the lamb in your air fryer's basket and cook at 380 degrees F for 15 minutes on each side. Divide everything between plates and serve.

Nutrition: calories 273, fat 13, fiber 4, carbs 6, protein 17

Ginger and Turmeric Lamb

Prep time: 15 minutes

Cooking time: 25 minutes

Servings: 4

Ingredients:

- 16 oz rack of lamb
- 1 teaspoon ginger paste
- ½ teaspoon ground ginger
- ½ teaspoon salt
- ½ teaspoon ground paprika
- ¼ teaspoon ground turmeric
- 1 tablespoon butter, melted
- 1 teaspoon olive oil

Directions:

1. In the mixing bowl mix up ground ginger, ginger paste, salt, ground paprika, turmeric, butter, and olive oil. Then brush the rack of lamb with the butter mixture

and put it in the air fryer. Cook the rack of lamb for 25 minutes at 380F.

Nutrition: calories 229, fat 14.2, fiber 0.2, carbs 0.6, protein 23.2

Parmesan Lamb Cutlets

Preparation time: 5 minutes

Cooking time: 30 minutes

Servings: 4

Ingredients:

- 8 lamb cutlets

- A pinch of salt and black pepper 3 tablespoons mustard

- 3 tablespoons olive oil

- ½ cup coconut flakes

- ¼ cup parmesan, grated

- 2 tablespoons parsley, chopped 2 tablespoons chives, chopped

- 1 tablespoon rosemary, chopped

Directions:

1. In a bowl, mix the lamb cutlets with all the ingredients except the parmesan and the coconut flakes and toss well. Dredge the cutlets in parmesan and

coconut flakes, put them in your air fryer's basket and cook at 390 degrees F for 15 minutes on each side. Divide between plates and serve.

Nutrition: calories 284, fat 13, fiber 3, carbs 6, protein 17

Mint and Rosemary Lamb

Prep time: 2 hours

Cooking time: 35 minutes

Servings: 2

Ingredients:

- 12 oz leg of lamb, boneless
- 1 teaspoon dried rosemary
- ½ teaspoon dried mint
- 1 garlic clove, diced
- ½ teaspoon salt
- ¼ teaspoon ground black pepper
- 1 teaspoon apple cider vinegar
- 1 tablespoon olive oil

Directions:

1.   In the mixing bowl mix up dried rosemary, mint, diced garlic, salt, ground black pepper, apple cider vinegar, and olive oil. Then rub the leg of lamb with the spice mixture and leave for 2 hours to marinate. After

this, preheat the air fryer to 400F. Put the leg of lamb in the air fryer and sprinkle with all remaining spice mixture. Cook the meal for 25 minutes. Then flip the meat on another side and cook it for 10 minutes more.

Nutrition: calories 382, fat 19.6, fiber 0.4, carbs 1.1, protein 47.9

Mixed Veggies

Prep time: 10 minutes

Cooking time: 5 minutes

Servings: 4

Ingredients:

- ½ cup cauliflower, diced

- ½ cup zucchini, diced

- 1/3 cup cherry tomatoes, chopped

- ¼ cup black olives, chopped

- 3 oz halloumi cheese, chopped

- 1 tablespoon olive oil

- ½ teaspoon chili flakes

- ½ teaspoon dried basil

- ½ teaspoon salt

- Cooking spray

Directions:

1.   Put the diced cauliflower in the air fryer pan. Spray them with cooking spray and then add zucchini. Preheat the air fryer to 395F and put the pan with vegetables inside it. Cook the vegetables for 5 minutes. Then shake them well and transfer in the salad bowl. Add cherry tomatoes, black olives, chopped halloumi, chili flakes, basil, and salt. Then add olive oil and mix up the anti-pasta.

Nutrition: calories 125, fat 25.8, fiber 0.9, carbs 2.8, protein 5.2

Balsamic Zucchinis

Preparation time: 5 minutes

Cooking time: 20 minutes

Servings: 4

Ingredients:

• pounds zucchinis, sliced

• 2 ounces feta cheese, crumbled 1 tablespoon parsley, chopped

• ¼ cup olive oil

• 2 tablespoons balsamic vinegar 1 teaspoon thyme, dried

• A pinch of salt and black pepper

Directions:

1. In a pan that fits your air fryer, mix the zucchini slices with the other ingredients except the cheese and toss. Sprinkle the cheese on top, introduce the pan in the fryer and cook at 400 degrees F for 20 minutes. Divide between plates and serve as a side dish.

Nutrition: calories 203, fat 9, fiber 3, carbs 6, protein 5

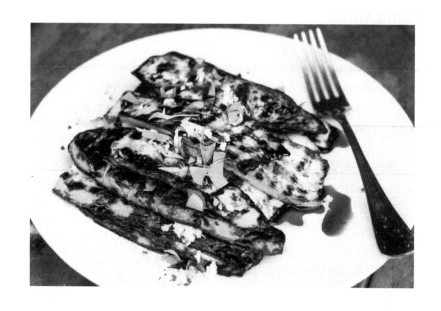

Leeks and Spring Onions

Prep time: 10 minutes

Cooking time: 6 minutes

Servings: 4

Ingredients:

- 1 cup spring onions, chopped

- 3 leeks, sliced

- 2 oz Parmesan, grated

- 1 egg, beaten

- ½ teaspoon ground black pepper

- 1 teaspoon dried parsley

Directions:

1. Preheat the air fryer to 400F. Combine all the ingredients inside and cook for 6 minutes.

2. Divide between plates and serve.

Nutrition: calories 91, fat 4.5, fiber 2, carbs 6.6, protein 6.9

Basil Zucchini Noodles

Preparation time: 5 minutes

Cooking time: 15 minutes

Servings: 4

Ingredients:

- 4 zucchinis, cut with a spiralizer 1 tablespoon olive oil

- 4 garlic cloves, minced

- 1 and ½ cups tomatoes, crushed Salt and black pepper to the taste 1 tablespoon basil, chopped

- ¼ cup green onions, chopped

Directions:

1. In a pan that fits your air fryer, mix zucchini noodles with the other ingredients, toss, introduce in the fryer and cook at 380 degrees F for 15 minutes. Divide between plates and serve as a side dish.

Nutrition: calories 194, fat 7, fiber 2, carbs 4, protein 9

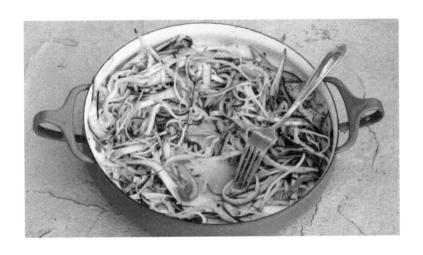

Zucchini Fritters

Prep time: 10 minutes

Cooking time: 10 minutes

Servings: 4

Ingredients:

- 2 zucchinis, grated
- 4 oz Blue cheese
- 1 egg, beaten
- 1 tablespoon flax meal
- 1 teaspoon dried cilantro
- ¼ teaspoon salt
- ¼ cup spring onions, chopped
- 1 teaspoon olive oil
- 3 oz celery stalk, diced
- 1 tablespoon coconut flour

Directions:

1.   Crumble Blue cheese and mix it up with grated zucchini. Add egg, flax meal, dried cilantro, salt, spring onions, diced celery stalk, and coconut flour. Then stir the ingredients with the help of the spoon until homogenous. Make the fritters and sprinkle them with olive oil. After this, preheat the air fryer to 400F. Place the zucchini fritters in the air fryer and cook them for 5 minutes. Then flip the fritters on another side and cook for 5 minutes more or until they are golden brown.

Nutrition: calories 164, fat 11.6, fiber 2.8, carbs 6.9, protein 9.6

Coconut Zucchini Gratin

Preparation time: 5 minutes

Cooking time: 25 minutes

Servings: 4

Ingredients:

- 4 cups zucchinis, sliced

- 1 and ½ cups mozzarella, shredded 2 tablespoons butter, melted

- ½ teaspoon garlic powder

- ½ cup coconut cream

- ½ tablespoon parsley, chopped

Directions:

1. In a baking pan that fits the air fryer, mix all the ingredients except the mozzarella and the parsley, and toss. Sprinkle the mozzarella and parsley, introduce in the air fryer and cook at 370 degrees F for 25 minutes. Divide between plates and serve as a side dish.

Nutrition: calories 220, fat 14, fiber 2, carbs 5, protein 9

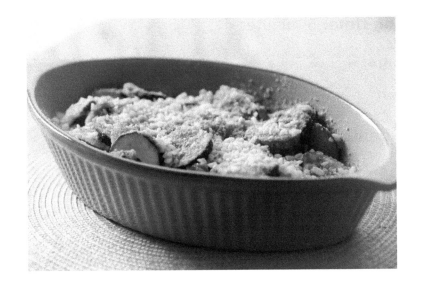

Ricotta Asparagus Mix

Prep time: 10 minutes

Cooking time: 5 minutes

Servings: 4

Ingredients:

- 11 oz asparagus, trimmed
- 5 oz gouda cheese, grated
- 1 teaspoon ground paprika
- ¼ teaspoon salt
- 1 teaspoon olive oil
- ¼ tablespoon ricotta cheese

Directions:

1.   Slice the asparagus and sprinkle it with ground paprika, salt, and olive oil. Then place it in the air fryer mold and top with grated gouda cheese and ricotta cheese. Preheat the air fryer to 400F. Insert the mold in the air fryer basket and cook the meal for 5 minutes.

Nutrition: calories 155, fat 11.1, fiber 1.8, carbs 4.2, protein 10.8

Parmesan Artichokes and Cauliflower

Preparation time: 5 minutes

Cooking time: 20 minutes

Servings: 4

Ingredients:

* 1 tablespoon olive oil

* 1 cup cauliflower florets 2 garlic cloves, minced

* ½ cup chicken stock

* 1 pound artichoke hearts, chopped 1 tablespoon parmesan, grated

* 1 and ½ tablespoons parsley, chopped Salt and black pepper to the taste

Directions:

1.   In a pan that fits your air fryer, mix all the ingredients except the parmesan and toss. Sprinkle the parmesan on top, introduce the pan in the air fryer and cook at 380 degrees F for 20 minutes. Divide between plates and serve as a side dish.

Nutrition: calories 195, fat 6, fiber 2, carbs 4, protein 8

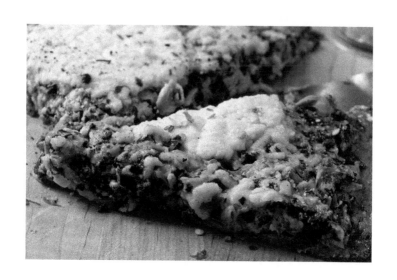

Butter Zucchini Noodles

Preparation time: 5 minutes

Cooking time: 15 minutes

Servings: 4

Ingredients:

•   1 pound zucchinis, cut with a spiralizer 2 tomatoes, cubed

•   3 tablespoons butter, melted 4 garlic cloves, minced

•   3 tablespoons parsley, chopped Salt and black pepper to the taste

Directions:

1.   In a pan that fits your air fryer, mix all the ingredients, toss, introduce in the fryer and cook at 350 degrees F for 15 minutes. Divide between plates and serve as a side dish.

Nutrition: calories 170, fat 6, fiber 2, carbs 5, protein 6

Dill Bok Choy

Prep time: 20 minutes

Cooking time: 5 minutes

Servings: 2

Ingredients:

* 6 oz bok choy

* 1 teaspoon sesame seeds

* 1 garlic clove, diced

* 1 tablespoon olive oil

* 1 teaspoon fresh dill, chopped

* 1 teaspoon apple cider vinegar

Directions:

1. Preheat the air fryer to 350F. Then chop the bok choy roughly and sprinkle with olive oil, diced garlic, olive oil, fresh dill, and apple cider vinegar. Mix up the bok choy and leave to marinate for 15 minutes. Then transfer the marinated bok choy in the air fryer basket and cook for 5 minutes. Shake it after 3 minutes of cooking. Transfer the cooked vegetables in the bowl and sprinkle

with sesame seeds. Shake the meal gently before serving.

Nutrition: calories 84, fat 8, fiber 1.1, carbs 3, protein 1.8

Bacon Green Beans Mix

Prep time: 15 minutes

Cooking time: 13 minutes

Servings: 4

Ingredients:

- 1 cup green beans, trimmed

- 4 oz bacon, sliced

- ¼ teaspoon salt

- 1 tablespoon avocado oil

Directions:

1.   Wrap the green beans in the sliced bacon. After this, sprinkle the vegetables with salt and avocado oil. Preheat the air fryer to 385F. Carefully arrange the green beans in the air fryer in one layer and cook them for 5 minutes. Then flip the green beans on another side and cook for 8 minutes more.

Nutrition: calories 167, fat 12.3, fiber 0.9, carbs 2.6, protein 10.5

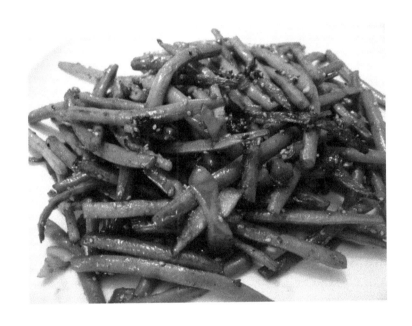

Garlic Endives and Scallions

Preparation time: 5 minutes

Cooking time: 20 minutes

Servings: 4

Ingredients:

- scallions, chopped

- garlic cloves, minced 1 tablespoon olive oil

- Salt and black pepper to the taste 1 teaspoon chili sauce

- endives, trimmed and roughly shredded

Directions:

1. Grease a pan that fits your air fryer with the oil, add all the ingredients, toss, introduce in the air fryer and cook at 370 degrees F for 20 minutes. Divide everything between plates and serve.

Nutrition: calories 184, fat 2, fiber 2, carbs 3, protein 5

Peppers Cups

Prep time: 10 minutes

Cooking time: 12 minutes

Servings: 12

Ingredients:

- 6 green bell peppers

- 12 egg

- ½ teaspoon ground black pepper

- ½ teaspoon chili flakes

Directions:

1. Cut the green bell peppers into halves and remove the seeds. Then crack the eggs in every bell pepper half and sprinkle with ground black pepper and chili flakes. After this, preheat the air fryer to 395F. Put the green bell pepper halves in the air fryer (cook for 2-3 halves per one time of cooking). Cook the egg peppers for 4 minutes. Repeat the same steps with remaining egg peppers.

Nutrition: calories 82, fat 4.5, fiber 0.8, carbs 4.9, protein 6.2

Chives Spinach Frittata

Preparation time: 5 minutes

Cooking time: 20 minutes

Servings: 4

Ingredients:

- 1 tablespoon chives, chopped 1 eggplant, cubed

- 8 ounces spinach, torn Cooking spray

- 6 eggs, whisked

- Salt and black pepper to the taste

Directions:

1. In a bowl, mix the eggs with the rest of the ingredients except the cooking spray and whisk well. Grease a pan that fits your air fryer with the cooking spray, pour the frittata mix, spread and put the pan in the machine. Cook at 380 degrees F for 20 minutes, divide between plates and serve for breakfast.

Nutrition: calories 240, fat 8, fiber 3, carbs 6, protein 12

Mozzarella Rolls

Prep time: 15 minutes

Cooking time: 6 minutes

Servings: 6

Ingredients:

- 6 wonton wrappers
- 1 tablespoon keto tomato sauce
- ½ cup Mozzarella, shredded
- 1 oz pepperoni, chopped
- 1 egg, beaten
- Cooking spray

Directions:

1. In the big bowl mix up together shredded Mozzarella, pepperoni, and tomato sauce. When the mixture is homogenous transfer it on the wonton wraps. Wrap the wonton wraps in the shape of sticks. Then brush them with beaten eggs. Preheat the air fryer to 400F. Spray the air fryer basket with cooking spray. Put

the pizza sticks in the air fryer and cook them for 3 minutes from each side.

Nutrition: calories 65, fat 3.5, fiber 0.2, carbs 4.9, protein 3.5

Parmesan Muffins

Preparation time: 5 minutes

Cooking time: 15 minutes

Servings: 4

Ingredients:

- 2 eggs, whisked Cooking spray

- 1 and ½ cups coconut milk 1 tablespoon baking powder

- 4 ounces baby spinach, chopped 2 ounces parmesan cheese, grated 3 ounces almond flour

Directions:

1. In a bowl, mix all the ingredients except the cooking spray and whisk really well. Grease a muffin pan that fits your air fryer with the cooking spray, divide the muffins mix, introduce the pan in the air fryer, cook at 380 degrees F for 15 minutes, divide between plates and serve.

Nutrition: calories 210, fat 12, fiber 3, carbs 5, protein 8

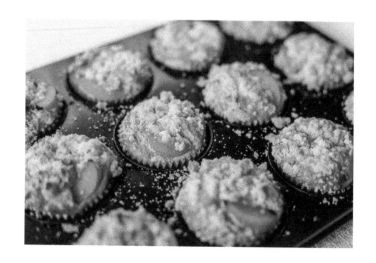

Cheese Eggs and Leeks

Prep time: 5 minutes

Cooking time: 7 minutes

Servings: 2

Ingredients:

- 2 leeks, chopped

- 4 eggs, whisked

- ¼ cup Cheddar cheese, shredded

- ½ cup Mozzarella cheese, shredded

- 1 teaspoon avocado oil

Directions:

1. Preheat the air fryer to 400F. Then brush the air fryer basket with avocado oil and combine the eggs with the rest of the ingredients inside. Cook for 7 minutes and serve.

Nutrition: calories 160, fat 8.2, fiber 7.1, carbs 12.6, protein 8.6

Peppers Bowls

Preparation time: 5 minutes

Cooking time: 20 minutes

Servings: 4

Ingredients:

- ½ cup cheddar cheese, shredded 2 tablespoons chives, chopped A pinch of salt and black pepper
- ¼ cup coconut cream
- 1 cup red bell peppers, chopped Cooking spray

Directions:

1. In a bowl, mix all the ingredients except the cooking spray and whisk well. Pour the mix in a baking pan that fits the air fryer greased with cooking spray and place the pan in the machine. Cook at 360 degrees F for 20 minutes, divide between plates and serve for breakfast.

Nutrition: calories 220, fat 14, fiber 2, carbs 5, protein 11

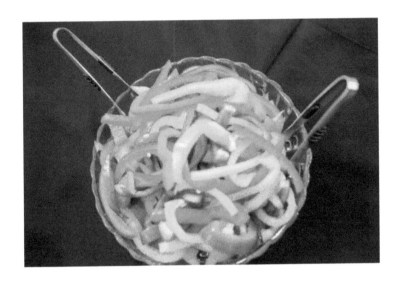

99

Bacon Eggs

Prep time: 15 minutes

Cooking time: 5 minutes

Servings: 2

Ingredients:

- 2 eggs, hard-boiled, peeled

- 4 bacon slices

- ½ teaspoon avocado oil

- 1 teaspoon mustard

Directions:

1. Preheat the air fryer to 400F. Then sprinkle the air fryer basket with avocado oil and place the bacon slices inside. Flatten them in one layer and cook for 2 minutes from each side. After this, cool the bacon to the room temperature. Wrap every egg into 2 bacon slices. Secure the eggs with toothpicks and place them in the air fryer. Cook the wrapped eggs for 1 minute at 400F.

Nutrition: calories 278, fat 20.9, fiber 0.3, carbs 1.5, protein 20

Balsamic Asparagus Salad

Preparation time: 5 minutes

Cooking time: 10 minutes

Servings: 4

Ingredients:

- 1 bunch asparagus, trimmed 1 cup baby arugula

- tablespoon cheddar cheese, grated 1 tablespoon balsamic vinegar

- A pinch of salt and black pepper Cooking spray

Directions:

1. Put the asparagus in your air fryer's basket, grease with cooking spray, season with salt and pepper and cook at 360 degrees F for 10 minutes. In a bowl, mix the asparagus with the arugula and the vinegar, toss, divide between plates and serve hot with cheese sprinkled on top

Nutrition: calories 200, fat 5, fiber 1, carbs 4, protein 5

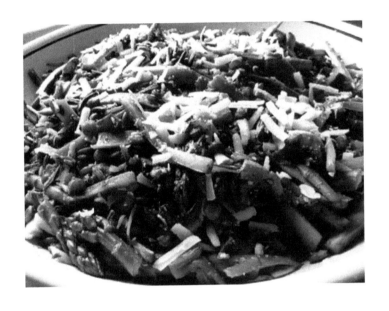

Cheddar Pancakes

Prep time: 10 minutes

Cooking time: 7 minutes

Servings: 2

Ingredients:

- 2 tablespoons almond flour
- ¼ teaspoon baking powder
- 1 teaspoon Erythritol
- 1 teaspoon cream cheese
- 1 teaspoon butter, melted
- 2 eggs, beaten
- 1 bacon slice, cooked, cut into halves
- 1 Cheddar cheese slice
- 1 teaspoon sesame oil

Directions:

1. Make the pancake batter: in the mixing bowl mix up baking powder, almond flour, Erythritol, cream cheese, and 1 beaten egg. Preheat the air fryer to 400F.

Then line the air fryer with baking paper. Pour ¼ of the pancake batter in the air fryer in the shape of pancake and cook for 1 minute. Then flip the pancake on another side and cook for 1 minute more. Repeat the same steps with the remaining pancake batter. You should get 4 pancakes. After this, brush the air fryer basket with sesame oil. Pour the remaining beaten egg in the air fryer and cook it for 3 minutes at 390F. Cut the cooked egg into 2 parts. Place the 1 half of cooked egg on the one pancake. Top it with 1 half of the bacon and second pancake.

Nutrition: calories 374, fat 31.7, fiber 3, carbs 7, protein 18.7

Green Beans Salad

Preparation time: 5 minutes

Cooking time: 20 minutes

Servings: 4

Ingredients:

•	cups green beans, cut into medium pieces 2 cups tomatoes, cubed

•	Salt and black pepper to the taste 1 teaspoon hot paprika

•	1 tablespoons cilantro, chopped Cooking spray

Directions:

1.	In a bowl, mix all the ingredients except the cooking spray and the cilantro and whisk them well. Grease a pan that fits the air fryer with the cooking spray, pour the green beans and tomatoes mix into the pan, sprinkle the cilantro on top, put the pan into the machine and cook at 360 degrees F for 20 minutes. Serve right away.

Nutrition: calories 222, fat 11, fiber 4, carbs 6, protein 12

Mini Almond Cakes

Preparation time: 10 minutes

Cooking time: 20 minutes

Servings: 4

Ingredients:

- 3 ounces dark chocolate, melted

- ¼ cup coconut oil, melted 2 tablespoons swerve

- 2 eggs, whisked

- ¼ teaspoon vanilla extract 1 tablespoon almond flour Cooking spray

Directions:

1. In bowl, combine all the ingredients except the cooking spray and whisk really well. Divide this into 4 ramekins greased with cooking spray, put them in the fryer and cook at 360 degrees F for 20 minutes. Serve warm.

Nutrition: calories 161, fat 12, fiber 1, carbs 4, protein 7

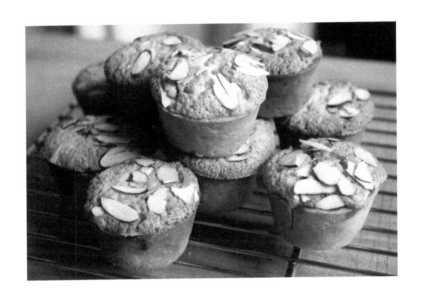

Lightning Source UK Ltd.
Milton Keynes UK
UKHW020641220621
385951UK00004B/51